THE
PARALYZING TRUTH

Finding Strength and Hope in the Midst of Tragedy and Grief

BY
Judith Sherwood

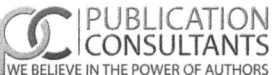

PO Box 221974 Anchorage, Alaska 99522-1974
books@publicationconsultants.com, www.publicationconsultants.com

ISBN Number: 978-1-63747-012-1
eBook ISBN Number: 978-1-63747-022-0

Library of Congress Number: 2023935439

Copyright © 2023 Judith Sherwood
—First Edition—

All rights reserved, including the right of reproduction in any form, or by any mechanical or electronic means including photocopying or recording, or by any information storage or retrieval system, in whole or in part in any form, and in any case not without the written permission of the author and publisher.

Manufactured in the United States of America

DEDICATIONS

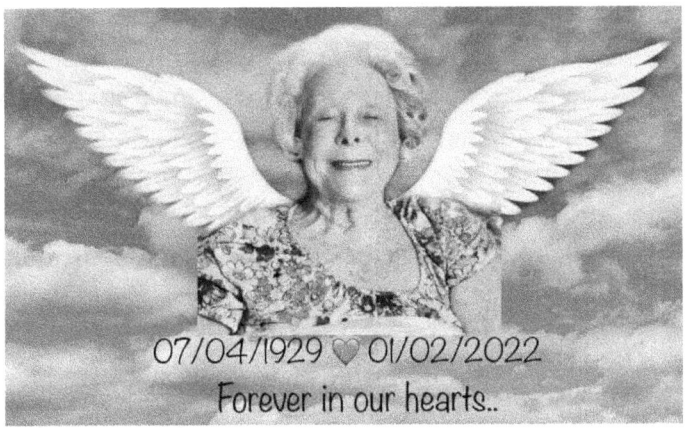

In loving Memory

Mom - who has always been an inspiration to us all with her unconditional love and unfailing faith to get through even the most difficult times in her life. We miss you so much, it hurts. You will forever be in our heart.

I dedicate this Book to .....

Jesus - *Immanuel* - He has been our strength every step of the way, continuously there for us, and listening to all our prayers.

Shaylynn - My daughter, who moved in with her family and helped me care for Mom since 2011. I could not have done this without you. It was a long 12 years of caregiving and there were times it got so hard for both of us, but we managed to help each other through it all. You have been a blessing. Love you! Paul Jones thank you for always being Moms night and shining armor, she always appreciated you for making her transfer easy by swooping her up out of bed, she appreciated you so much for making it less of a chore and it made her want to get up more. Love you!

Sterling & Jena - My son, thank you for making the video and putting all the pictures and music together for the celebration of life, love you. Jena, my daughter-in-law, as always, I appreciate your love and support and all you do for us. Love you both!

To all our family and friends that have supported Mom and us throughout her journey with prayers, encouragement via Facebook, phone calls, cards. We are forever grateful. Mom truly felt blessed.

PREFACE

The *Paralyzing Truth* is about how a tragedy turned into a triumph with the help of our Lord and Savior Jesus Christ. It demonstrates how faith was the guiding force which not only got my Mother through her ordeal, but also all of us through as well.

The inspiration and motivation for me to write this book is my Mom, Olga Kleinertz. I became her caregiver back in 2009 when she walked into the hospital for an out-patient procedure for pain relief... and never walked out.

This book details all she had to endure as a result. Though she would never regain the ability to walk and be independent again, she always managed to give a smile and go with the hand life had dealt her. And she did it with such grace and acceptance.

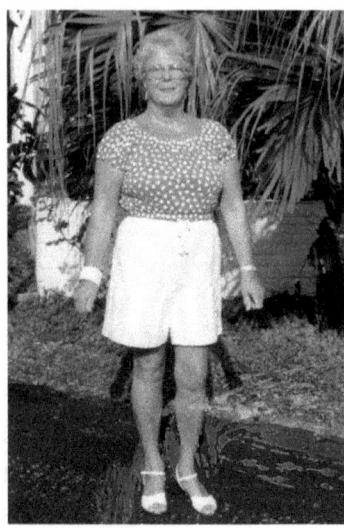 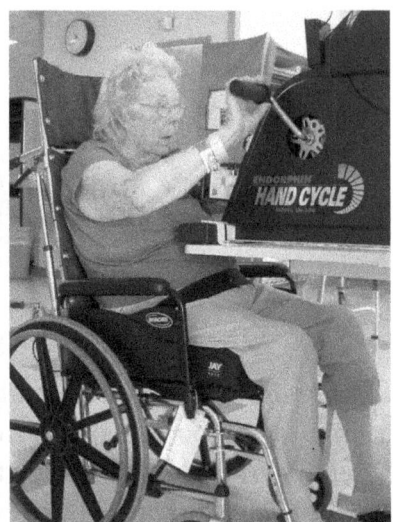

Being her caregiver for the next 12 years, and seeing first-hand what her life was now like day-in-and-day-out, became a deep inspiration for me. As her caregiver I often experienced being tired, exhausted, and, honestly, struggled on days to keep going. And this, at times, to the very point of tears. Yet, it was here the patient, my Mother, who would console me!

As you will read, I had the privilege to care for her, along with with my daughter, in order to fulfill her ultimate wish, that she be able to reside in her home until the day she passed.

There had been many challenges along the way. Often it seemed like we were, indeed, "at the end." But through the grace of God, prayers, and our own advocating for

Mom, she got through those many close calls. The truth is, she reached the point where she wasn't expected to live another year, let alone *two* more years... but she did. And in your reading, you will see how Mom had been followed on Facebook in all of this by so many who shared in her entire journey.

Since Mom passed away on January 2, 2022, my life has been turned upside down. I awoke one Saturday morning some months afterward, and just started typing on the computer.

Before I knew it, I had completed and was naming chapters, as my former journaling turned into this book.

My intent is to share it with not only family and friends, but with all of Moms Facebook followers. Beyond that, is the desire to encourage anyone who is going through some tough times and can, thus, be inspired by our story. I hope they will see even though Mom never walked again, or gained her independence, she was able to be an overcomer. God met her right where she was at and gave her a strength that "superseded all understanding." There is *nothing* that we faced during the last 12 years of My Mom's life that God couldn't handle and get us through.

So, may God be *your* strength through the storms in your life, and may He fill you with His peace, love, and joy. In Jesus name, Amen.

TABEL OF CONTENT

Preface   5

Chapter 1: The appointment   11
Chapter 2: The day the music died   14
Chapter 3: The elephant in the room   18
Chapter 4: At the shore   22
Chapter 5: Home is where the ramp is   26
Chapter 6: Goodbye independence   30
Chapter 7: The men in her life   34
Chapter 8: Tripping on hospital visits   38
Chapter 9: Bring me my teeth cup   43
Chapter 10: Hospice-tality   47
Chapter 11: Our last christmas   51
Chapter 12: Church family and faith   55
Chapter 13: New year's eve   59
Chapter 14: This isn't goodbye, it's see you later   64
Chapter 15: Celebration of life   69

CHAPTER 1
THE APPOINTMENT

It was as if it were yesterday: In 2009 our mother walked into the hospital for an epidural for pain management... and never walked out. A day that none of us will forget. It was, almost appropriately, the morning of April 1st, I was at Mom's house for my usual morning visit to have breakfast and I would usually stay for the remainder of the day. Mom was on the phone making a call to a doctor's office trying to get an appointment. She was on hold when I asked her what she was doing. She replied she was trying to get an appointment for an epidural. She wanted it done before her up-coming vacation to Ocean City in July. She wanted her neck, often in constant ache, to be pain free so she could enjoy her vacation. She had an epidural the year prior with great success and was hoping for the same results.

When she was finally taken off hold, the doctor's office let Mom know they could squeeze her in for an appt. on Friday to begin the first round of a set of three injections that would take place over a period of time. I kept hearing Mom repeat a number of times into the phone saying, "This Friday? Friday?"

So the appointment was set for Friday April 3rd, just two days later from that phone call to make the appointment. {I emphasize *two days* later, which you will understand why shortly).

I also heard my Mom talking about some medications. Although she handled all of her own affairs, I did remind her of her newest one that she had been put on within the current year. It was the result of her having stents put in. The new drug was Plavix. So she told the doctor's office she was on Plavix, which was something new, and of which they were not aware. They directed her to NOT take the Plavix the morning of the now scheduled procedure. I know this because I was seated there as Mom repeated it back to them to confirm she understood.

As Mom hung up the phone, I asked her who she was talking to? Of course I am bound to silence and can't say in this book his name but we can call him Dr. Negligence, "Dr. N" for short. For my own peace-of-mind, I asked her *again* what was said about the Plavix and she proceeded to say the doctor said *not* to take it the day of the procedure. As an after-thought, I did ask Mom about Aspirin. But she said they didn't say anything about that. So, just to be sure, I told her not to take *anything* that morning and just bring meds with her.

At the time, it didn't occur to any of us to question the doctor, none of us were experts on Plavix. We did know it thinned the blood. But as far as how the procedure might conflict with the Plavix, we trusted the doctor and medical staff knew what they were doing. After all Mom had been to this doctor a number of times before for the epidural and trusted him.

The appointment was now all set! Mom was excited to get the procedure done, as she had done the previous year, but this year in order to be pain free for her vacation.

On the Morning of April 3rd, I was watching my grandson at the time, I packed him up in the car, picked up my Mom, and dropped her off at Outpatient Medical Facility. My sister, Terry, would be picking her up once the procedure was done.

Mom was always the type of person that never wanted to inconvenience anyone. As much as I wanted to go in and wait with her, she knew I had my grandson to watch while my daughter was at work. "Honey, I don't need you to wait; you've got Austin to watch. I will see you later after the procedure."

With that, I left to go about my day. Little did any of us know that this appointment was about to change the rest of her life-and our lives-forever.

CHAPTER 2
THE DAY THE MUSIC DIED

All I remember that day was I was summoned to come up to the hospital. As I recall, my sisters Terry and Diana were there. When I arrived, Mom was lying in bed saying she could not move her legs. She kept hitting her legs saying, "I can't feel my legs." My Mother could not move them at all. As Mom described what had happened, she said she also had chest pains, and then her legs went into spasms. She repeated, "I can't feel my legs."

This all took place in recovery after the procedure. The Doctor had left already for the day. So the doctor was called by the nurse. When she got off the phone she came over and said to us the doctor wanted Mom to get up and into the chair as preparation to get ready to go home.

Mom with the look of panic, begged them not to put her on her feet. She said, "I can't feel my legs; I am going to fall!!" The nurse merely responded, "It's going to be ok honey."

Yet, sure enough... the Fall!

Judith Sherwood

As soon as the three nurses attempted to stand Mom up the chest pains immediately began again. At the same time, and in the words of Emeril, "BAHM!!!"- she fell to her knees. Mom might as well have been invisible as her pleas went completely ignored.

Back into bed she went. Once again Dr N was called, and instead of coming back to assess the situation, *over the phone* he directed Mom be admitted. That's it, just admitted.

I stayed as late as it was allowed, and got back to the hospital as early the next morning as I could get in. I was told Mom had a rough night. She couldn't urinate and the build-up of urine was becoming extremely painful. She ended up with a catheter being inserted just prior to my arrival.

The previously AWOL Dr. N arrived early in the morning. At Mom's bedside he seemed to be feeling her leg... exploring it. He then pricked her leg to see if there was a reaction of pain. All the while it seemed to me that there just didn't seem to be any urgency on his part. My mother expressed to him that, "Maybe there is something really wrong here, because I can't stand up at all!

I mean really? Mom walks into the hospital and she can't walk out and he shows no signs of urgency when he shows up the next day? I wonder what he had planned after Mom's procedure, because his lack of attention changed all our lives forever.

Not long afterwards Mom's bone doctor, "Dr. M," came in. It was with this doctor the urgency began. From Mom's description of what she was experiencing, he quickly surmised what was wrong and immediately had her taken down for an x ray.

When he came back in, the x-ray results in hand, he explained what was happening. He told us Mom had a hematoma. She had been bleeding "inside," causing intense pressure on her spine. And, because of the delay, there was now only a small window of opportunity to get that compression off of there.

Otherwise, she would be permanently paralyzed.

I don't want you all to miss this important fact: Because Mom wasn't off her Plavix for the *required* five to seven days prior to her procedure, she started bleeding in recovery at the injection site. And this probably almost immediately after the procedure. This caused a clot of blood to form causing a hematoma that compressed her spine. In turn, this caused the chest pain and leg spasms that left her unable to feel her legs.

Keep in mind that from the time of the procedure to the next day's accurate diagnosis, Mom's hematoma had been compressing her spine now for over 20 hours. So in reality, the small window of time opportunity to prevent permanent paralysis... went out the window, you might say.

Dr. M did immediately rush Mom down to surgery to remove the hematoma. But sadly, the damage had already been done. And over the next few days that reality began to sink in.

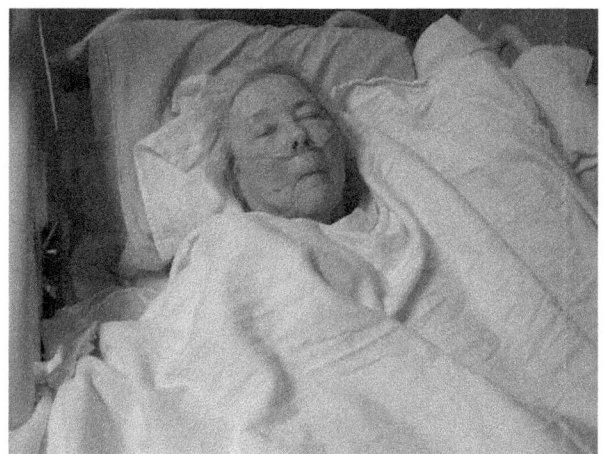

CHAPTER 3
THE ELEPHANT IN THE ROOM

Up to this point, here is what we knew....
1. Mom wasn't taken off her Plavix for the proper allotted five to seven days that her epidural steroid injection called for.
2. She was only told to *not* take the Plavix on the day of the procedure.
3. In the nurse's notes it said Mom was asked if she took *Plavix that morning* and Mom said "No."
4. In recovery Mom experienced chest pains and spasms in her legs. She also could not feel her legs anymore, all of which she expressed to the nurses attending her.

This pretty much sums up the obvious. See if you can spot the Elephant...

Mom arrived at the hospital and checked in. She was sent over to the area where she would be getting her shot.

She waited until she was called. The nurse took Mom in the back and they talked a little bit as she took Mom's blood pressure and pulse. All the while the nurse asked Mom questions about her medical history.

She then asked Mom what medications Mom was currently on. Mom gave her a list she purposely brought of those medications. According to Mom, the nurse put that list on the clip board.

Specifically, the nurse asked Mom *When did you last take your Plavix and Aspirin?* Mom answered and told her she did not take them that morning, the day of procedure, as directed. Mom then saw the nurse write something down on the clipboard she was holding at which point she gave Mom the clipboard with the consent form on it. Mom glanced at it then signed and dated it. Then the nurse proceeded to tell Mom to get her clothes off and change into her hospital gown.

There was no other discussion from the nurse about the forms Mom signed, nor about Plavix, Aspirin, or any of her other medications. Mom got the gown on and just waited until finally another nurse came in to get her and wheel her down to the operating room. Mom never saw the other nurse that took her medication list and asked her when she last took Plavix.

Mom later stated that Dr. N came into the operating room and that was the first she saw him that morning. It really had been the first she had seen Dr. N in over a year. He never asked her about her medications, specifically Plavix or Aspirin.

Mom was in the operating room with Dr N for about 15 minutes prior to the procedure beginning. As expected, she still doesn't remember anything after receiving the anesthesia. The next thing she remembers is waking up and being very groggy... and still in the operating room. Yet she was able to sense that there was now no pain. It was then a nurse wheeled her back into the recovery room.

Mom says she remembered her breasts began feeling weird and then she had this horrible pain from her back around to her chest. That eventually stopped, but it was followed by a horrible pain in her legs, even though the legs themselves felt numb.

HMMMMM! Care to venture a guess as to what was happening at this point? The oversight of the medical protocols regarding Plavix was the undetected Elephant in the room, literally. The Hematoma was beginning to set in. The "Can't feel my legs" expressed to the nurse should have raised Red Flags. I mean, *How was this missed?!!?* It should have been obvious!

It is well known Lidocaine wears off in 6 hours... or less. So, if it was the cause of the numbness, this Mom's lack of feeling in her legs should have worn off no later then 9:00 p.m. That *something* was wrong should have been obvious at this point, especially considering Mom still had no feeling in her legs... and worse, still couldn't stand up.

All I can say is Captain Obvious, you have been demoted to Dr. Negligence. Seriously, at this point he could *have-should* have-at least ordered an x-ray. But Dr. N had departed the hospital. He was gone for the rest of the day... and night, after Mom's procedure.

Mom doesn't remember much more after this part because she ended up in the Intensive Care Unit (ICU}. She was sent to the ICU, because it was determined she needed a blood transfusion. Who made the decision for that, we still don't know. But *somebody* knew something was wrong.

Everything then became a blur. It was unbelievable; we were all in shock. We were not even sure Mom was even going to survive. This, literally, was taking the life out of her... and us.

I never prayed so hard in all my life for her recovery.

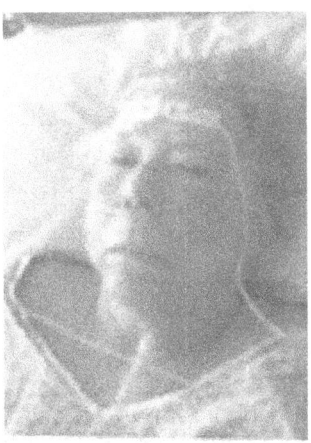

ICU

CHAPTER 4
AT THE SHORE

Mom made it through ICU and after that she had to go to Shore Rehab for, of course, "rehabilitation." She was feeling very defeated and frustrated at the time. She still had no feeling in her legs and could not use her right arm, which she used for *everything*. Mom was also still on a catheter, because she as yet couldn't urinate on her own.

The Rehab worked with Mom and taught her how to start using her right hand again. But in the end, she taught herself how to eat left-handed, because she couldn't use her right hand like she used to. Further, they taught Mom how to sit up properly in bed when getting ready for transfer into her chair, as well as how to assist during the process of that transfer.

Mom continued to have pain in her arm and in the one leg she couldn't move, but could feel. She would still get those spasms and just have really bad intermittent pain. Mom would continually tell the Rehab staff, "I want to walk again! I want to be myself again!" But she was not recovering; there was so much she still could not do.

As an example, Mom's bladder wasn't working at all. Being on a catheter turned out to be a condition that remained for the rest of her life. She also had no control over her bowels; they too were not working anymore either. This meant she needed help from us extracting them at times. (I know... too much information). But this is what we were dealing with! The result of all this, Mom was left needing to wear diapers... all the time.

As it turned out, Rehab was *brutal* for Mom. They used what they called a "standing machine." Using this contraption, they would strap Mom into it and lift slowly in increments to get her to a standing position. The problem was when they would stand her up, her blood pressure would drop. She would get dizzy or nauseous and so she could not be up long. Inevitably, they would have to put her down.

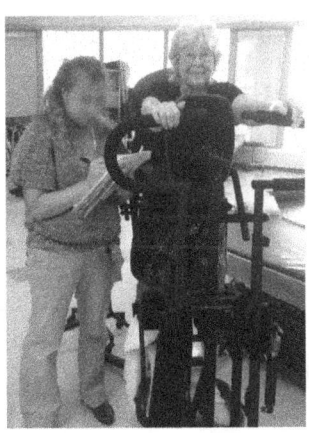

The other painful issue she had to endure was if they put her in a position where she had to use her shoulders. In that procedure her rotator cuff would tear into her shoulders, which really could not support her weight. This always increased her fear of falling.

Shore Rehab was intense to say the least. My heart just ached for what my Mother was going through. Not only having to be on a catheter with a bag, she would have bowel accidents during her physical therapy and she felt embarrassed. I mean, I can understand her feeling that way, and she would have to stop therapy.

During this time we were also getting a better understanding of what had occurred on the day of Mom's procedure. Plavix, paired with the injection, caused internal bleeding, a "hematoma," which compressed, intensely pressed on, Mom's spine for over 20 hours. This pretty much crushed the nerves affecting her bladder, her bowels, her arms, her hands, her legs. (Need I go on?} Rehab for Mom at that point, as far as I was concerned, was like polishing a brass railing on a sinking ship! It was useless!

From Shore Rehab Mom went to Rose Garden, allegedly another place of rehabilitation, but more accurately, a nursing home. As I remember, she was there about six weeks. Rehab was definitely less intense then Shore Rehab. They tried a lot of exercises, again practiced how to move from a bed to a chair, how to eat, and how to use her hands especially her right hand.

And it was there she got a motorized wheelchair.

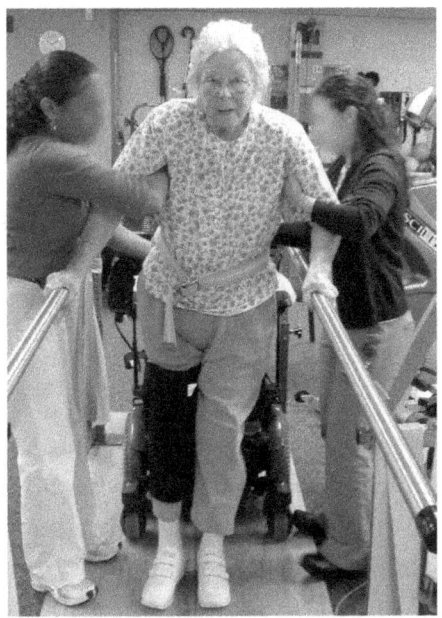

CHAPTER 5
HOME IS WHERE THE RAMP IS

Now that Mom was home, she needed her home to accommodate her needs. Family came and built a ramp outside so her wheelchair could get in and out of the house. Her bathroom had to be remodeled to fit a shower chair into which she could be wheeled. What an ordeal that shower chair was!

To transfer Mom into that chair, which had six clips that had to be shuffled around to put the back down, as well as to unhook the base in order to move out the step... Phew!! I would always work up a sweat! If I thought *my* showers were long, the process for Mom was just overwhelming, to say the least.

Further, she needed a special kind of bed... and she now needed a van to accommodate her wheelchair in order to get to and from the various doctors. Everything Mom needed, right down to the payment of caregiving, supplies or whatever else, most of it all came from her own wallet. The ramp was for cost of materials only; thank goodness for that blessing!

When Mom first came home, she paid for an aide for the first three months. The cost was about $ 5,000 a month. Mom couldn't get help through insurance until she depleted all her funds in her annuity, from which she drew a budgeted amount, monthly. Mom was quickly depleting her money for this care plan. As a result, I started caring for Mom in September of 2009.

For convenience, and to be with her at all times, I moved into her home. As the workload became progressively harder, in 2011 my daughter moved in (along with her family) to help me. Caring for Mom was a lot of work and I sure appreciated the help. With this added help from my daughter, we were able to cut the cost of having any full-time aide. This helped preserve as much as we could of Mom's money and still be able to cover our living expenses.

Everything was being done with the intent to grant Mom's wish of remaining in her own home. Mom especially loved her bedroom. We had come to dub it the

Pepto Bismol Room, because that is what the color of her room reminded us of. She really did love pink!

And because this would be her living quarters as well, I made sure to set everything up to make it as easy as possible for Mom to function: Right down to her bed table, which provided drawers for her to access her personal things... and to hide her candy-Mom *did* have a sweet tooth!

I also placed a garbage pail within her reach, and ensured her access to the ceiling fan control, the light fixture via remote control, and television remotes. I even had a call bell for her to click when she wanted me. Eventually, I put a camera in her room allowing me to look in at her through the night. I even brought a mirror to sit in front of her plate so she could actually see where her food was at in order to grab it. You would be surprised how difficult it is, especially being paralyzed, to get yourself upright enough to see your plate!

That was just all the physical things. We had yet another thing to tackle, and that was all the emotions that started leaking out and surfacing now that she was home. All of this was part of her, and us, getting used to her "new normal." And, as part of this acclimation process, you go through every scenario in your mind back to that fateful day, hoping to make sense of it all.

What you need to know about Mom is she does not linger in the self-pity pool. She most definitely knows how to embrace what hand life has dealt her, and how to make the best of it. Mom, no matter how she feels emotionally, will always have compassion and smiles to give away. It might be hard at times to know what's behind her smile, but she never burdens anyone with self-pity. This is because she is so genuine and readily gives of herself and heart to all. I have always been just so in awe of her strength, tenacity, perseverance, and unconditional love, but never more so than through this ordeal. Mom always had a loving spirit that just radiated from her that made it so easy to love her in return. And she was so easily loved, indeed by all.

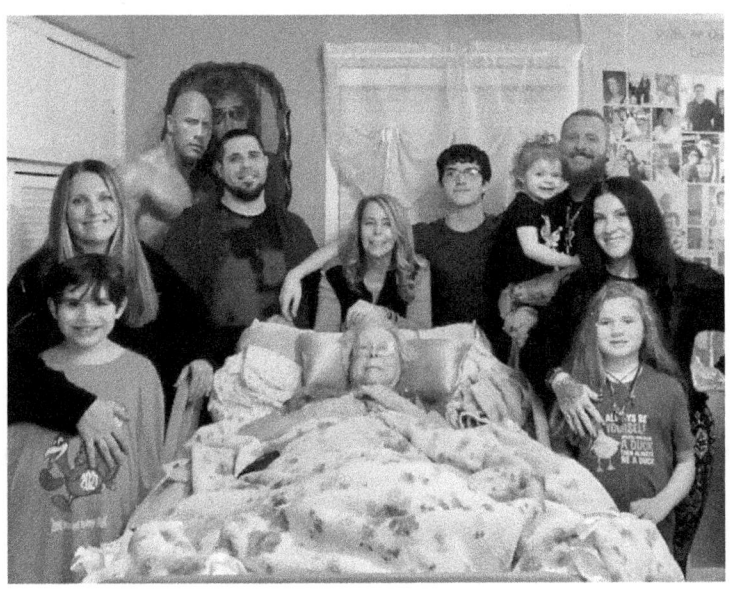

CHAPTER 6
GOODBYE INDEPENDENCE

It is important to understand what it was like to be a round-the-clock caregiver. This included, but was not limited to the following:

- Cooking - Breakfast, Lunch, and Dinner
- Keeping the water jug filled at all times throughout the day, organizing and providing medications at their proper times, periodic blood pressure monitoring.
- Bathing, complete "in the tub," or as-needed "wash downs" Changing clothes, not just daily, but also as often "as-needed"
- Toileting, which included changing diapers (and "clean-up) and bed pads, both as-needed
- Changing the catheter once a week, or as-needed

Emptying the catheter bag, multiple times a day

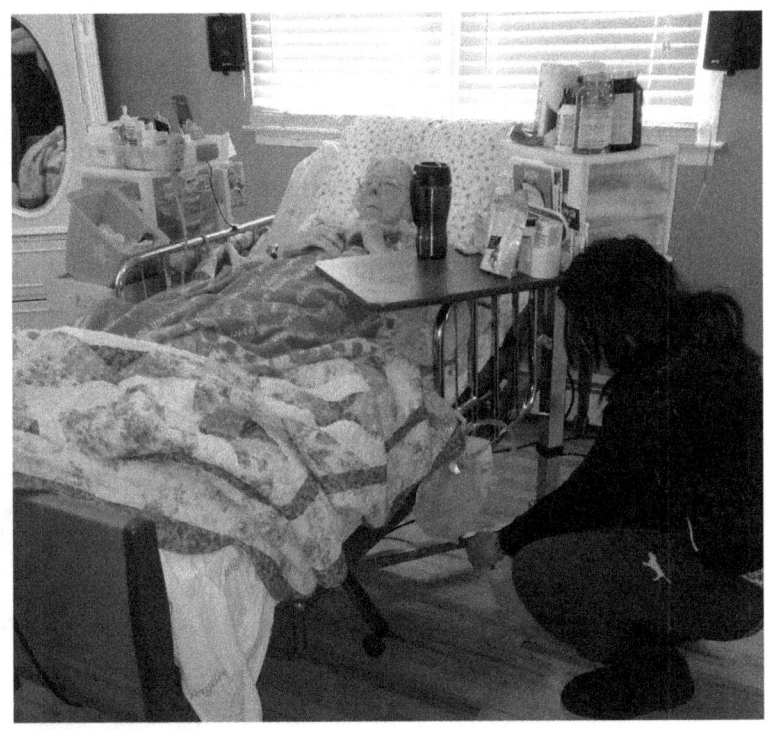

All the laundry

Exercising Mom's legs Moving her from side to side
Transferring out, and back into bed
Running her to doctor appointments

Running errands, picking up scripts, and other "driving" chores, wound care should she hurt herself or get a bed sore

Providing Companionship, such as watching television with her,
conversations-meaningful or otherwise-and lots of hugs and love
Food, and "other" shopping, house cleaning.
Providing Mom with anything she needs that she literally could not get up out of bed to do for herself.
Continuously, pulling her up in bed when she would slide down. Changing positions in bed.

My Mother was asked these series of questions by the attorney handling our case:

1. *How do you feel about Judy being your nursing aide?* "It breaks my heart that she has to do this for me. She should be enjoying her own life, but now she has become my nurse. I really appreciate what she is doing, but I feel bad for her that she has to do this. It is also hard because I changed Judy's diapers and now she is changing mine. Had this not happened, I would be able to do everything for myself."
2. *Is it difficult for you being dependent upon others?* "Yes. It is incredibly difficult. I do not like it. I do not have any ability to do anything on my own. I cannot do anything without someone helping me.
3. *Is this how you envisioned living your 80s?* "Not at all!"

If you never been a caregiver for someone who is paralyzed, I want you to know it is very challenging. The physical demands alone of transferring, dressing, having to pull the patient up in the bed quite often when they have slid down are wearing. Your body especially starts to feel it over a long period of time.

Then there is the emotional part. Caregiving is a whole other ball game (which I will cover in my next book, to help others like myself that have had to care for a loved one). It is not easy for both the patient having lost their independence and become dependent, as well as for the loved one caring for them. It truly is an emotional rollercoaster for all involved.

But I promise you this, I would not change a thing... It was an honor to be there for my Mom and care for her. She has always been there for me, not only when I was child, but also as an adult. She has been the best mother and grandmother any of her family could have ever asked for.

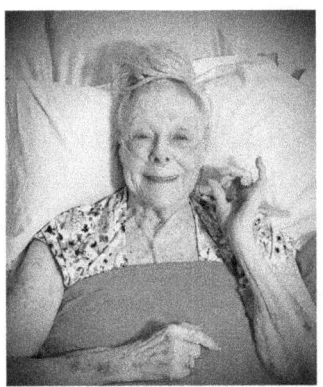

CHAPTER 7
THE MEN IN HER LIFE

I call this *The Men In Her Life* because in Mom's isolation, we really did as much as we could to make her smile. We knew her First Guy was Elvis Presley. Mom has always been a huge fan of this 1950s heartthrob. And as Mom always enjoyed life with gusto, when she had opportunities to do things with us, she wouldn't hesitate to dive in.

Mom got an invite from my sister, Terry, to go to Nashville. This trip would include seeing so many country stars, even getting their autographs. But it would especially include a tour through Graceland, Elvis' home. They had a blast!

I think my brother, Craig, was the one who got us all hooked on Elvis. He always watched Elvis' movies and would sing around the house to his songs. Sadly, my brother died in 2017 from Sepsis; just another thing Mom - and all of us - had to go through. Rest In Peace Craig. We love and miss you so much!

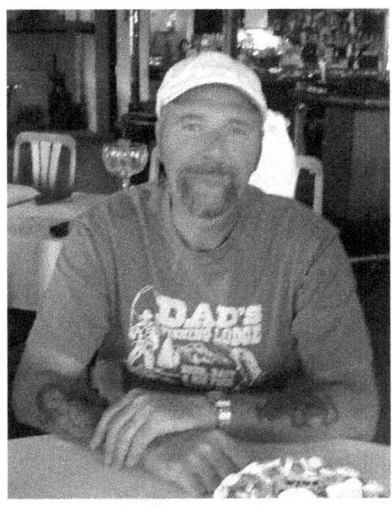

On one Christmas Eve we surprised Mom with an Elvis Impersonator. He came to our home to sing and entertain her, though I will say we *all* enjoyed the performance! Our home was full of people, not only family, but many friends as well. And the Ocean Star, our local newspaper, took pictures and printed them along with an article about Mom's "show." It was the best time *ever!*

My Mother loved the television show, *The Voice*. She would watch it without fail. Her favorite judge was Blake Shelton. Mom probably could not name one song he sings, she just knew him from *The Voice*. But she loved his humor, and she especially liked his looks! When she saw him sing on *The Voice* and other Country Music Television (CMT) award shows, she just loved his voice. I honestly think she was daydreaming that he was singing *to her!*

Another favorite of hers was Dwayne Johnson. We watched a couple of his movies one night and she was hooked on him from that night on. Could it be his obvious talent as an actor? His witty humor? Well besides the obvious, it was that he was bald and, thus, handsome. Yup! Mom loved bald men!

So, with all of this in mind, for her birthday I got Mom a *life-sized* cutout figure of Blake Shelton. At the same time, my sister got one of Dwayne Johnson. and They remained with her in her room, close to the bed, ever since. In fact, they even attended her Celebration of Life after she passed. Though I did make the (unsuccessful) attempt to get an actual meet-and-greet from both men, Mom was just as happy with her life-like cutouts of her favorite men.

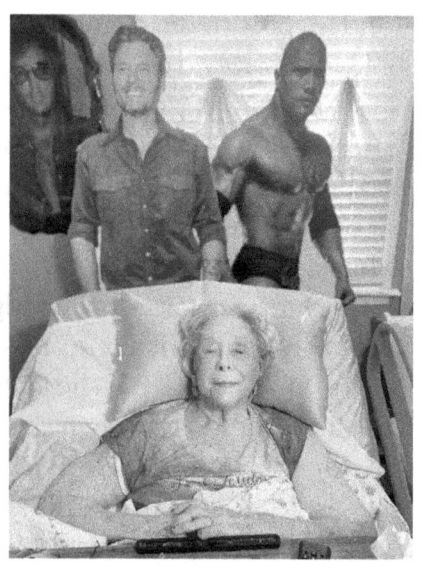

Oh, I can't forget about Simon Cowell from America's Got Talent (AGT). She absolutely ADORED him!!! If I had a dime for every time she mentioned Simon during the show each time we watched it together, well I would be RICH! I can't remember why we didn't get a life-sized board of Simon. Maybe at the time I couldn't find one. Who knows? But Mom *never* missed seeing him on AGT. He too was one of the men in her life!

CHAPTER 8
TRIPPING ON HOSPITAL VISITS

I cannot tell you how many times Mom has been in and out of the hospital. Before the Covid pandemic hit, Mom's hospital room always looked like an assembly line. Family was always up there. We would set up a table to play card games. Most of the time we had music playing. The nurses loved coming into her room. And most of the time she lucked out and had a private room.

Mom was always surrounded by some really wonderful nurses and aides. In fact, Mom would have some pretty good-looking aides that would come in to wash her. I was there early one morning and Mom had just finished breakfast. She said the aide was coming in to wash her. Not long afterwards, in comes this good-looking male aide. Mom immediately starts pushing the covers off, pulling up her gown. I started laughing and said, "Geesh Mom! Play a little hard to get! At the very least, make him take you to dinner first!" Well, we all laughed so hard, we were in tears. Humor really is the best medicine.

There was this one aide, he happened to be an associate pastor, he was always on Mom's floor and had to tend to her. He would get us to surround Mom's bed and then we would all pray with her. It was beautiful. One other time a nurse took such a liking to Mom, she surprised her with a birthday cake. Truly was amazing!

Mom had so much love. I advocated for her when she was in the hospital. I was up there every day making sure she ate. I even tended to her with toileting when the nurses were busy so Mom didn't have to wait and sit in a dirty diaper. I would also always monitor her medications when she was in the hospital. Even to the extent of having them take her off some pill of which I was not originally aware, but one that made her lethargic. Yes, having someone to advocate for you especially in the hospital-is so important.

Five years prior to Mom's passing, we had discussed with good intentions, to eventually have Hospice Care at home. But, at the current moment, we knew Mom wasn't ready for that. She was still able to go to her doctor appointments, and so, not being totally bedridden, she wanted proactive care.

In early January 2021, Mom's lungs filled with fluid. This time she had to go to the hospital via ambulance. Because of the Covid pandemic, they would not let me in. This was devastating to me. Mom had never really been alone at the hospital before, with the exception of visiting hours ending. She had always been surrounded by family during her hospital stays. Further, I was her advocate and had *always* been involved in her care. I felt so isolated, yet, try as I may, they would not let me in there.

After sitting in the parking garage calling the hospital too many times to count, I was getting frustrated thinking, *How can this be? I am her caregiver!* I felt I was living in a nightmare right then. I was crying so hard I thought I was going to pass out. I was drained... But I never stopped praying.

I finally received a call from the hospital and was told I was able to come in to see the doctor and Mom. When I arrived on her floor and initially walked past her room to talk with the doctor, I could see she was on a Bipap Machine.

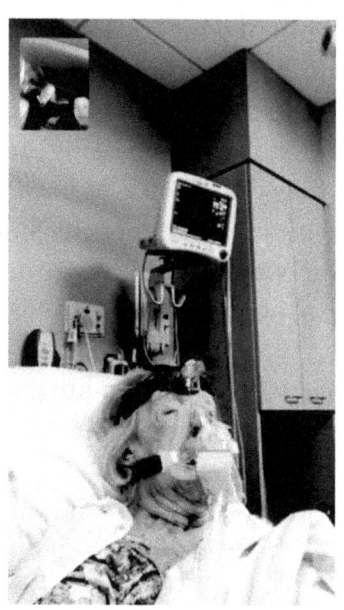

I knew this was used to assist those with troubled breathing.

It was then the doctor and assisting nurse asked me about Hospice. I immediately said no, that was *not* a consideration. I was told my Mom would not be coming home. Her lungs were filled with fluid, and her oxygen level was dangerously low. I responded they had yet to treat her. First, make an attempt to save her life. Give her that chance at least. "You don't know my Mom. She does not want to die here!" The nurse looked at me and said, "Honey, your Mom isn't *ever* coming home." I replied, "Well then, I will have to pray for a miracle."

With that, I got up to go and see Mom before I had to leave. It was hard for her to talk. She looked up at me as I told her they would not let me stay. She managed to say, "They won't?" I said "No, they won't. But I *will* get you home. You keep fighting. Everyone will be praying for you. She nodded a *yes*. I then hugged her and the nurse made me leave.

I didn't immediately leave the parking garage. I sat there crying and praying. Between sobs, I reached out to everyone I could think of for prayers. I posted on Facebook and asked for prayers from everyone who had been following Mom's journey on there from the beginning. I reached out to our church family. I wasn't sure I was ever going to leave the hospital parking garage.

It was hours later, well after dark and nearing 10:00 p.m. when I got a call on my cell phone. It was my kids. They were very worried about me. My daughter anxiously said to me, "Mom, you are worried about your Mom and we are worried about *ours.*" It was then I decided to start for home.

I love you Sterling and Shaylynn.

CHAPTER 9
BRING ME MY TEETH CUP

That same night I went home, I got another call from the hospital. They wanted to put Mom on hospice, and they were calling to get my permission. It felt like the Never-Ending Hospice Train. Well, I wanted off that crazy train.

Frankly, I was at the point I wasn't sure how much more I could take. My eyes were slits, I wasn't allowed to be up there with Mom to see what was going on, and I knew my Mother, She wouldn't want it. So, I said *no.* And I emphatically asked them *not* to call me again on this issue. I reiterated they needed to actually treat her and give her a chance to get better.

The rest of the night was a blur for me.

The next morning the nurse called me again. She began by apologizing. I know you said no to hospice, but they want me to ask you again if you will re-consider it today for your Mom." All I could say at that point was that I would not make any decision unless they let me up to see my Mom. The nurse said ok, and arranged for me to come up.

I said a silent prayer after I hung up. I went tearfully to my daughter and said, "They are letting me in to see Nanny; I will keep you posted. I can't make any decisions until I see her and know what's going on."

About an hour or so later, as I was getting ready to go up to the hospital, the nurse called me again. But this time she had a different request. Your mom would like you to bring her teeth cup when you come." I instantly rejoiced! This was music to my ears! I *knew* she was going to be okay. And I was in tears.

A teeth cup is what Mom kept her false teeth in and she didn't have her teeth in when they took her to the hospital. My Mom was thinking *longterm!*

When I got up to the hospital, Mom was sitting up in bed talking and smiling. The nurse who had called me earlier that morning about hospice approached me and said...

"When I took the BiPap machine off so your Mom could take some of her meds, your Mom began talking up a storm. And when I checked, her oxygen level it was staying way up, so I kept it off."

I then Face-timed my daughter so she could actually see her Nanny and be surprised. Boy was she!

The doctor came in and told me that my Mother's lungs were clear and he was releasing her so she could go home. I thought I was done with the "waterworks," but I wasn't. We definitely thanked everyone that prayed for her, and thanked God for his mercy and grace for Mom.

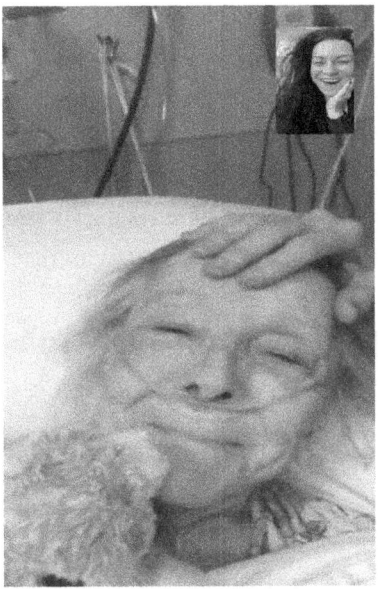

I reflected on how, during so many of the trips to the hospital, Mom was treated as if she were senile. To be fair to them, however, they didn't know her. This is why I find it important for medical staff, including doctors, to get to know their patient through the family members. No one knows that patient better, especially a family member who is the constant caregiver; the one who cares for them day in and day out.

As a result of this trip to the hospital, it was at this point that Mom made an irrevocable decision. Given the circumstance now with Covid restrictions on family, those that prevented family members from visitation, she made it known she did not want to go to the hospital anymore...

ever. I explained in detail what that meant. She said she fully understood. She made it clear, *emphasized* it, that when it was "her time to go," she wanted *it* to be "at home" surrounded by family.

Truth be told, Mom had now reached the point where we could clearly see she was weak and her body was not cooperating with her anymore. It was now only a matter of time.

And we knew when Mom was ready, she would tell us...

CHAPTER 10
HOSPICE-TALITY

When we started with Hospice, I needed to change what we called it. I came up with *Comfort Care.* They would come in and bring us the Comfort Care Kit, with all the ingredients to keep Mom comfortable during the rest of her journey.

Notwithstanding the name change and its implied meaning, it took some time to come to a meeting of the minds.

You see they have *one* goal in mind and that's comfort. If there is a remote twinge of pain... give the morphine; if the patient was sleeping... don't wake them up to eat. So, there were a lot of things I did that made them look at me as if I had two heads. But I did them, nonetheless.

You see, I explained to them I would treat Mom as if she were "still living," not as if she were about to die. Most of them were not use to that perspective. I made it clear I would wake her up for meals, because she needed to eat. If she didn't want to, then I would let her go back to sleep. I would also keep her entertained, especially by her watching all her favorite television shows. This would provide her with something to look forward to each day.

Further, I would keep up with her pain meds that were working for her instead of the morphine which left her "groggy." In this way, she could continue to enjoy her family, especially grandkids, her shows, or any company who came to visit. Mom was comfortable with the care and treatments we provided, so we didn't change a thing. The Hospice workers got to see we enjoyed as much of our time together as we could, watching movies, laughing, playing Yahtzee, and having wonderful meals together.

It just was amazing the last year, a "Hospice year," that we had with her. Mom knew the Comfort Kit was always available and if she needed something - anything -- to keep her more comfortable, we would give it to her.

In the beginning I knew each time Hospice came in they would point out she has edema and it was only going to be getting worse as it moved up to her flanks. I am sure they believed I thought Mom was going to live forever. This was their way of a gentle reminder for me to do a reality check. And I knew they didn't think Mom was going to last as long as she did.

Each week the nurse came out she was pleasantly surprised at Mom's resilience. She would always praise us for the love and care Mom got, which she attributed to Mom's continued good days. Subconsciously, I guess I felt that Mom was going to be around forever. But I knew the sad reality. Yet, I was just hoping she would make it to 100, so she could be on the Today Show!

All I knew was, each day I intended to love my Mom like I was going to lose her that day. I was going to treat her as part of the living and enjoy as much as I could of our time together. The last year we had was more then we could ever ask for, we truly felt blessed. And all the while Mom had made it through moments that doctors, nurses, and Hospice staff would be left scratching their heads.

Love is so powerful; don't ever underestimate it. God had been so good to us. Our faith and hope was what made this bearable to accept what was happening. I really feel Mom's longevity was because she had great advocates in her corner to oversee her care. She was able stay in the home she loved, surrounded by family. And definitely her faith was what got her through a lot. We just tried to really make the worse days of her life the best days... to the best of our ability.

After a while, Hospice began to understand my mindset, and I theirs. They came to stop resisting my routine for Mom. I really think they were quite shocked and pleasantly surprised at Mom's strength and perseverance. And Mom was always a willing participant.

One time I had a dermatologist come to the home because Mom had some lesions on her legs and they were not looking so good. They continued to get bigger and were oozing a tad. The Doctor said it looked like Squamous cell, which can be cancerous. To make sure, he did remove them and had them tested. Sure enough, it was.

I remember the Hospice nurse asked me, prior to the results, if it was cancer, what would I do? Give her Chemo? I replied we just wanted to take care of the lesions that seemed to be getting out of control, that's all. I knew all-to-well that this type of cancer would take a long time to claim Mom's life, even though it was clear Mom's health had taken more of a decline.

Notwithstanding, we certainly didn't want Mom's wound to become infected. I know what the Hospice nurse was conveying: Why put mom through anything else. Mom knew the lesions were there, because I was caring for them. To have a better understanding, she wanted me to take a picture and show her. When I did, she didn't like what she saw. That's when I suggested contacting a dermatologist and seeing if he would come out to our home and examine her. Mom smiled, as she always did, and said okay. Done!

I wanted to allow my Mom to decide for herself, not only in this, but in how the rest of her journey would play out. I would guide her, but ultimately each decision was hers. I could understand that she wanted to feel she still had a say in her life...

She had lost everything else.

CHAPTER 11
OUR LAST CHRISTMAS

It was December 11. Mom was still feeling pretty good. In fact, she did one of her video talks on Facebook saying hello to everyone, thanking her Facebook family for all the love, prayers, and always being there for her. I got the white Christmas tree out and set it up in her room with all the lights and special ornaments we had personalized for that tree. The tree was propped up high enough for Mom to see and enjoy. She just loved it! It brought her so much cheer and warmth in her room. I loved getting Mom excited about Christmas.

Every night without fail her grandson, Austin, would come upstairs and hug his grandma and kiss her on the forehead. It became something she looked forward to every night that sincerely touched her. One particular night Mom was just so emotional, crying in his arms, and saying how much she was going to miss him, how much she loved him. She truly felt blessed to be able to stay home and be surrounded by her family.

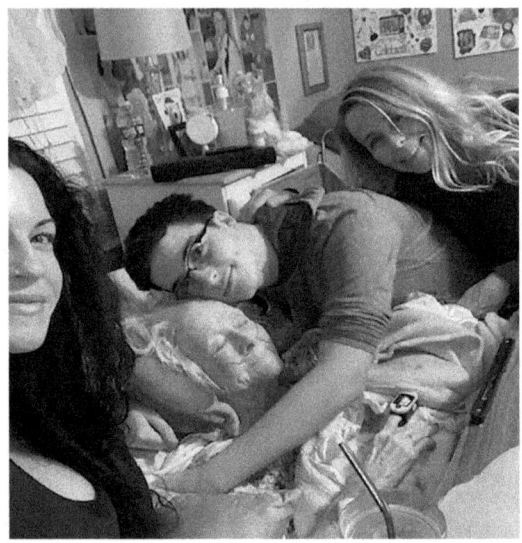

This December was a month that would be hard to forget: Covid hit. It started with me, ran through the house, and though we all tried to protect Mom, sadly she, nonetheless, did come down with it. We did everything we could to keep her comfortable during her illness.

Mom was already experiencing the edema. The buildup of fluids in her body was becoming very aggressive. She had been leaking out at the catheter insertion site, which was in at her stomach area. We knew the edema was working its way up to her lungs, but we were so grateful that it had this still-working release point.

But I could see the inevitable. Yet, I didn't want to acknowledge that; to actually believe what was really taking place. Worse, I had no one who could turn to me and say,

"This is the final countdown." I mean my Mom just always pulled through. I couldn't picture my life without her.

During this time, I did what I always had done and tried everything I could to keep her comfortable and help her get better. There were times in the past when Mom would gather us at her bedside and say I think this is it... then she would apologize if she didn't die.

We would all chuckle and say we were grateful that you didn't Mom. I just always thought when it *was* really time, she would let us know in a way that was more obvious; a way that was, frankly, staring us in the face.

That last Christmas morning together, we all went in with all her presents in-hand. She mustered up the strength to say *Merry Christmas*. And she smiled, as she always did. But there was something different this Christmas. I could tell her mind was going. She was present in body, feeble as it was, but her spirit was noticeably waning. And neither of us could find the courage to confront that.

I opened her presents for her as she was too weak, and still running a fever. She loved everything she got. The grandkids came in and opened the presents from her to them. I always made sure to shop for her to have gifts to give, because giving was always more of a joy for her then receiving.

This Christmas day she wasn't ready for her morning coffee and the little, white, powdered donuts she usually loved so much.

That morning... she just wanted to rest.

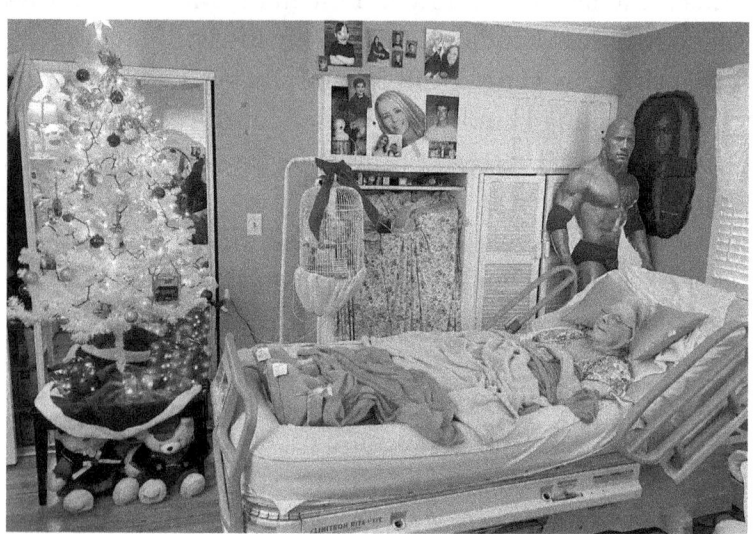

CHAPTER 12
CHURCH FAMILY AND FAITH

It was becoming so unbelievably difficult to face, seeing Mom day in and day out just lying in her bed. The only interaction she had with the outside world was when people would come to visit, or when any us who were caring for her would gather in her room to watch television or movies, or play music or games with her. The loneliness, at times, made her wish the Lord would come for her. It just tore me up inside.

She had grown weary of feeling sick and tired. I could only imagine what she was going through. But to see her still always readily give us a smile in spite of how she was feeling, just warmed my heart. It was indeed a testament to her very character.

I belonged to a Bible study with a wonderful group of women who always prayed for Mom and who were always reaching out to her. They would come over to dote on her, and we all would sing Mom's favorite song, "How Great Thou Art" with Mom singing right along with us. It was beautiful to see, and Mom enjoyed it so much, especially when we would all pray with Mom.

The Church had also been so supportive in other ways. They provided for our needs when help was required. From the spiritual, as described above, to the making of meals, which they and dropped off, and to even financial support. It was a comfort and a blessing during our difficult moments.

My other Bible study group always was there to pray for Mom. In fact, it was the first study group Mom had ever been to prior to her accident. There she had embraced getting to know the Lord better and making lifelong friends.

Mom and I had been baptized together when I was around 10 years old. It was a day I will never forget. I am so grateful that she gave her life to Jesus… that we both did. The blessings of that commitment never stopped for Mom.

As an example, there was a wonderful gentleman from church his name was Michael Matt who was a singer and played guitar in church. He reached out to Mom because he and his wife had seen all our posts sharing Mom's life's journey, which included how much she loved music. He wanted to bless Mom and he came to our home with all his equipment and sang his heart out to her. She had a smile the whole time and felt so special having her own mini concert.

There is something to be said for and experiencing a church family. Even when they don't know you personally, there is this unspoken union that takes place where you just want share with, and support, your "extended family."

Such kindness just strengthens one's own faith spiritually, as you see the unconditional love and acceptance. It creates in your heart a confidence, a God confidence, that you are loved. As Christians we all strive to be like Jesus. And when that is demonstrated through one's actions in the way they live, it is so inspiring.

Mom had her own personal relationship with Jesus. She prayed every night. Her heart was one with Him. At times we would pray together and I loved listening to her child-like prayers, so innocent, so full of compassion. She had such a loving spirit that just radiated from her.

She also knew how to forgive, how to love unconditional, and how to show the compassion she felt. She made you feel good to be in her company, because she would always show you that things don't ever have to be perfect or right in your life to be happy. Mom was known for making good that current cliche of making lemonade out of lemons when life threw them at her. She was-and still is-truly my inspiration. In my mind, she has her heavenly Father's eyes, full of compassion, seeing the good in everything... in everyone.

So applicable is Isaiah 40:31,

> But they that wait upon the Lord shall renew their strength; they shall mount up with wings as eagles; they shall run, and not be weary; and they shall walk, and not faint.

That verse explains how she stayed so steadfast and strong through her entire ordeal. She was stronger than I could ever be in her shoes. She was truly amazing!

CHAPTER 13
NEW YEAR'S EVE

It was New Year's Eve. Mom was eating less. God bless her though; she had all her wits about her. She always knew what was going on, what she was saying.

Even at times, when she was dehydrated, the dehydration did occasionally make her confused where she would say off-the-wall things. This caused us all to laughter, even by Mom. She would hear what she was saying and wonder aloud, "What the heck am I talking about?" At times like that, I would just let her know it would pass. "You got yourself dehydrated and once we correct it, you will be fine." She would nod and say, "Okay."

One time she was saying there was a bird in her room and wanted us to catch it. She *swore* it was there. So rather than stress her out, we pretended to do just that. I used a fake bird I had gotten from the Dollar Store. We made a show of putting it in a cage that was in her room, made for her from someone at our church and with beautiful flowers around it. The whole thing was way too funny. When

Mom was feeling better, we told her all about it, and she just laughed.

This reminds me, one day I did get Mom a real bird. She named him Pretty Boy. We kept him on the table at her bedside and she would talk to him. She would call his name, "Pretty Boy," and then make kissing noises. She would do this every day multiple times a day.

Long story short, I now have her bird. She made me promise to take care of him once she was gone. He continues talking and saying everything my Mom would say to him. What a wonderful gift I have! This bird is a daily reminder of the joy this gift gave her... and now to us.

Getting back to New Year's Eve. I could see Mom was fretting. She wasn't saying much, but I could see she was "in a zone." She was fully aware of what was happening to her physically, and this night she was feeling that... silently.

I really didn't want to go out that night. I waited to see if Mom was going to ask me to stay home instead; as if she knew something I didn't. What might be hard for someone to understand is that, in the 12 years of caring for Mom, to my recollection I never missed a New Year's Eve with her. Some might see that as sacrificing a lot in my life, but I would rather spend that night and its moments while at her side when she needed me. It was something I so readily gave her.

But this year I asked my sister, Terry, to come sit with Mom for New Year's Eve. You see, my son, Sterling, was going to propose to his girlfriend this night at his New Year's Eve party. None of the party gatherers knew what was going to take place, and he wanted me there for the surprise.

I told Mom why I was going, because she loves when people say to her "Can you keep a Secret?" She *can't,* just so you know. But it does make her feel a part of something big when you do. I told Mom I loved her and that I would film it and show her when I got back home. She graciously nodded her head in acknowledgement.

I knew Mom well enough to know if she didn't want me to leave, she wouldn't tell me; she never wanted to impose. I truly was torn. It was a bittersweet moment.

It turned out to be, however, a wonderful escape. I was thankful to experience a moment of joy for my son. And I tried my best to only be in this moment of bliss and excitement for my son and his now, new fiancé. I *was* truly so happy for them both. But my Mom still weighed heavily on my heart.

The next morning, New Year's Day, I couldn't believe we are in the year 2022! Mom had reached a moment in the afternoon when she tried to speak, but she couldn't get the words out. This led her to start crying.

My heart was aching so much watching her frustration. I hugged her and tried to comfort her. I told her, "Mom I know it's frustrating not to be able to say words. I love you and I know you love us. I know your scared. We are going to keep you comfortable, and if you just rest you will feel better."

I actually started to believe what I was saying. Mom had come so close to death so many times, and yet she had defied it each time. Previously when she couldn't speak because she was dehydrated, a dose of pedialyte and some rest and the next day she was just fine. So I couldn't form the words to acknowledge that this time it could be "it."

As many times previously as Mom thought it was "her time" and gather us around her, I guess I might overlook *the* sign, even though it was staring straight at me.

Added to this was probably that I was in apparent denial. But to be safe, I summoned the rest of the family and they all came over for the day, staying well into evening.

Mom, as she now almost always was, rested during this day. We would periodically shift her on her side in order to pat her gently on her back. She was congested and doing this would break up any developing fluid or mucus.

Throughout all of this, Mom showed no signs of distress. But because she wasn't able to swallow her pills, we used a small dose of morphine, this for the first time, used in place of her pain medication in case she was in any discomfort.

My daughter and I did try to give her a sip of water. It appeared as if Mom did get a little sip, and so we both looked at each other and thought she is going to be okay. Denial is a frustrating road to travel. It's an emotional rollercoaster. We all kept telling her we loved her.

Her ex son-in-law was there that day too. When he said in his deep voice, "I love you Mom," her eyes opened wide as if startled, his voice was that piercing. Mom really loved him. She mouthed the words *I love you,* a confirmation we all got at different times.

By day's end Mom was still showing some signs of strength. Yet, we could see she was riding a current she could no longer resist. That night everyone said goodbye, with the encouragement they would see her again tomorrow.

With a little nod of her head, she showed us she was still with us... even though she couldn't speak.

CHAPTER 14
THIS ISN'T GOODBYE, IT'S SEE YOU LATER

It is now January 2nd, in the year of our Lord, 2022. The night before Mom had grabbed my hand and, because I knew her so well, held it as if to say/ *am scared*. At this point it was the only way she could communicate. She held on tight until she fell asleep.

But this is a new day and there seemed a new peace taking place with Mom. This was good, as everyone was back at the house early that morning.

We all wanted to make sure Mom was comfortable this day. My daughter and I knew from our experience with Mom over these years how her mouth would often get very dry. It was why she loved her water and always wanted it nearby.

But this morning she couldn't drink at all. So we tried to put ice chips up to her lips. But that didn't work either. With her eyes closed, she just shook her head *no.* We then decided to give her a half dose of morphine even though

Mom didn't appear to be in discomfort, we wanted to make sure that she wasn't feeling any pain.

We gave her a half dose of Morphine around 8:30 a.m. My concern with the morphine, as with all the pain medication she had taken over these past 12 years, was the possibility of painful withdrawal symptoms. I didn't want her to suffer any more than she already was.

After receiving the morphine, I checked Mom's blood oxygen level. I couldn't believe how good that level was through all this. And, thankfully, I could see she was peaceful.

I still can't process, much less adequately express, what I was going through. Because Mom had been in this predicament so many times before, I just expected it to turn out as it did in the past with her recovery. Those many recoveries had somehow conditioned me. As a result, I just honestly had never practiced for the moment for when "that time" really came. And it is also why I didn't recognize it when it did.

All morning we kept an eye on Mom, one or two of us going back and forth from the living room and kitchen where the family had congregated to Mom's bedroom. During this time her eyes remained always shut. I didn't want to speak or in any way wake her. I just wanted her to be peaceful, even if indeed she "passed." But I truly still felt we would get through this like we always did.

After my last trip into Mom's bedroom, I left to go to the bathroom, afterwards to grab a cup of coffee and sit at the kitchen table with everyone for a minute to gather my thoughts. It was then my other sister, Diana, had walked down the hall into Mom's room. After a moment I got up to do the same, when Diana came out of the room and said, "I think Mom just passed." I was stunned! I stammered, "What?" I could hardly catch my breath. I asked her, "What did you see?" She replied, "Mom just took her last breath and that was it. No distress. No floundering. No gasping."

My Mother went peacefully!

Even now I have to say *Praise God* for yet another prayer answered. Mom had been leaking fluid out her belly at the catheter entry site, so the fluid didn't have a chance to gather up into her lungs. God gave Mom and us the peaceful ascent into heaven we had long prayed for.

I on the other hand began to struggle with guilt. I had always pictured being there holding her in that final moment... and I wasn't. I was beside myself with grief. I couldn't let go of her; I couldn't leave the room; I didn't want to see Mom's bed *empty.* For that reason, I couldn't bring myself to even call the funeral parlor.

I believe Mom died about 10:30 a.m. But it was officially recorded by Hospice around 1:00 p.m. when they finally got there. My family was concerned about the delay. They especially wanted the funeral parlor notified. And I know everyone was worried about me, because I couldn't "let go." For the moment, though, I had to tune out everyone's concern as I was trying to deal with my grieving.

I had cared for Mom for these past 12 years. It had developed a relationship that was so close and so deep. I don't think anyone could have understood what I was feeling in that moment. All I knew is once the funeral parlor picked her up, it would be the last moment I would have to see her... and see her there in the room where I cared for her that entire time.

I just tried to process it all and take it in, and I had such a *hard* time. I literally couldn't stop hugging her as I cried. As crazy as it might sound, I found myself trying to put her pulse oximeter on her finger. It had been something I had done for *12 years*. Not seeing any readings tore me up even more.

Finally I made my peace and allowed the coroner to be called. I know I couldn't watch them come and take her away, so I curled up into a ball in my bed. I was numb trying to process this... as I cried long into the night.

I am not quite sure Mom would *not* have been able to let go peacefully if I was in the room with her. At least that is what I tell myself. Mom had always been worried about what would happen to me after she passed: What would I do; where would I live; how would I get through losing my best friend... I always told Mom what she needed to hear: That I would be okay. I have my church family. No one will see us "forced into the street."

The hardest part, I knew even then, I expressed to her," *I will miss you, Mom, s*o much!" And then I would reassure her, "But I will get through it by holding on to God's promises that we will see each other again." She would simply say, "Yes, we will." Then I would tell her, "Promise me you will wait until I get there." And with a twinkle in my eye I would add, "But do not ask God to come and get me before my time!" And we would both have a hearty laugh out loud.

I miss you Mom...
Until we meet again!

CHAPTER 15
CELEBRATION OF LIFE

Another bitter sweet day lies ahead of me now. An afternoon has been set aside to celebrate my Mother's wonderful life. And I do mean to *celebrate;* I want all who will attend to celebrate. I want these moments to celebrate all the essence of who Mom was. I want to feel the joy of her life. Even like we did each time in her presence as we entered her room during the past 12 years. shared by all to be obvious in her celebration.

Rick Young, who was our Bible study group leader, a group both Mom and I attended, had known Mom and visited her for years. He felt honored when I asked if he would speak at the Celebration on behalf of Mom. I asked him to do this since he knew so her well. I knew he would speak of her deep faith, truly representing the hope that she shared with everyone that she would be in the presence of the Lord at her death because of her faith. He truly did a wonderful job and Mom would have been crying right along with us. In his presentation he indeed captured the beauty of her life-long personality.

As part of the Celebration, my son, Sterling, put together a video that was shown to the attendees, both family and friends. In it, he showed a timeline of pictures of Mom, and with a fitting tribute at its end, recorded before her passing, of Mom thanking everyone for all their support and prayers. She closed with expressing her love to everyone present. All of this was beyond words, and so beautiful.

When I write that this Celebration captured Mom, it most certainly did. She would have loved it!! We had the life-sized cutouts of Blake Shelton and Dwayne Johnson there, of course! We brought her mechanical cat that simulated a real cat right down to the fur, purring, and, yes, *meowing,* which took place intermittently during my own speech.

Then there was the beautiful Memorial Cards of my Mom that my daughter, Shaylynn, developed that had beautiful, white, angelic wings, which made these Cards so special.

Our church family, along with other family and friends, provided the food, which made this Celebration all possible for us! We were so grateful for all the help from everyone with decorating the hall where the Celebration was held.

Did I mention we decided to have the Celebration at the nearby Moose Lodge? Why the Moose? Mom used to previously belong to it. We would go there quite often for their dinner specials and "occasionally" enter their pool tournaments. Few knew Mom was a bit of a pool shark. She would act like she didn't know what she was doing, but then she would magically be running the table!

There were a number of people who spoke at Mom's Celebration. So many beautiful words were spoken about her I barely made it through my own speech. I thanked everyone for being an on-going support for Mom during her journey. I expressed how grateful I was for Facebook, because it had allowed a window into Mom's life, into all our lives, these past 12 years of ups and downs together. I let everyone know how thankful we were for them embracing that journey with us and how Mom truly felt all their love and support. She really felt blessed and even like a celebrity at times.

I related how it was such a comfort of support for all of us involved in her care, and not just for Mom. She really enjoyed reading the beautiful cards, often with personal comments, of the many prayers, compliments, encouragements and just sharing others' joyful moments with her. It was uplifting to see people describing Mom in those writings using words like adorable, beautiful inside and out, special, kind, caring, sweet lady, amazing, fighter, a star, strong, precious woman, remarkable woman, and the list goes on and on. Someone even wrote, "Olga, your grace and gratitude in life is an inspiration to me!"

From all of this, what we will carry in our hearts forever is Moms strength, unconditional love, her smile that she so readily gave no matter how she was feeling, and all the wonderful inspirations expressed to describe Mom. These will always be the mark she left behind in all of our hearts.

The last years have not been easy for Shaylynn and I, being her caregivers. And though we have heard from time to time Mom expressing how lucky she felt to have us in that role, I can truly say, *we* were the lucky ones. In that, we now have the comfort and blessings to reflect and know that we were able to make the worse days of her life the best days. To the best of our ability, we provided a reason for her to keep going. It was such an honor to care for someone who was so selfless throughout her life. One who gave and loved unconditionally... truly the best Mom, Grandmother, relative, and friend anyone could ask for.

As seen in the video, if Mom were able to be here at her own Celebration, I know she would want to say thank you to everyone from the bottom of her heart for all your love and support you have given her throughout her journey. Because of that, you all gave her a reason to be alive. And she would express how God helped her through it all and gave her hope for the promise of eternal life, a deep held belief of her faith, to which she looked forward.

On behalf of our loving Mother, we want to end by sharing this hope with you.

> *For this is how God loved the world: He gave his one and only Son, so that everyone who believes in him will not perish but have eternal life.*
> (John 3:16).

Salvation doesn't come from our good deeds or by doing anything special; it is a free gift from God just because

He loves us so much. We need to acknowledge our sins, which require a Savior, and believe that Jesus is God's Son and that very Savior. Then we need to submit to Him as Lord, ruler of our lives.

If you are ready to begin that journey of faith and share in the same hope Mom shared with us all, we invite you to say this prayer to begin your life of faith and hope with Christ.

Father God,

> I come to you and you alone, for my salvation, I confess my sinfulness to you. I ask you to forgive me for Jesus' sake. I promise to put my trust in your Son Jesus from now on and I ask your help in doing it. I ask you to come into my heart and life, and make me your child according to your promise. I ask for the free gift of eternal life and for the free gift of your Holy Spirit. I ask you to let me know that I am really saved. I thank you Lord Jesus for saving me.

I ask all this in the name of Jesus, Amen

Know that, in doing this prayer, you too have now joined in Mom's Celebration of Life!

* * *

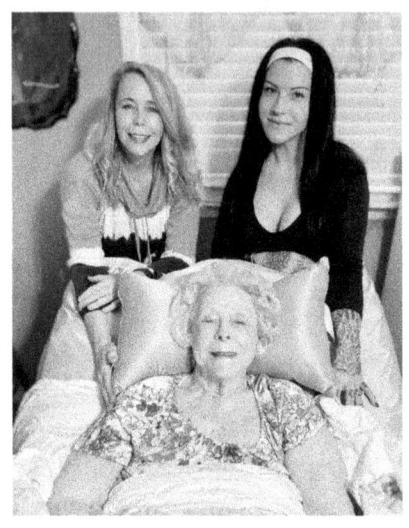

There is Hope inside of Grief

Romans 8:18
Yet what we suffer now is nothing compared to the glory He will reveal to us later.

Our Hearts miss you so much it hurts.

Our minds continue to flood with the wonderful memories of you.

What gives us hope and joy is remembering where you are and that we will be together again for eternity one day.

Forever in our Hearts until we meet again xoxo

www.ingramcontent.com/pod-product-compliance
Lightning Source LLC
Chambersburg PA
CBHW060852050426
42453CB00008B/957